Healthy Spine from Metabolism

Effective Ways for Coping with Back Pain and Sciatica

Introduction

Do you wish to optimize your back health so you can live a more fulfilled and independent life for the long haul?

Have you been experiencing unexplained back discomforts, reduced mobility, or excruciating pains like sciatica?

If you've answered YES to any or all of the questions above, then:

You are in luck because this book will show you exactly how to cope with back pains naturally, deal with sciatica and optimize the health of your spine without relying on pain medication!

According to research,[1] back pain is one of the most common reasons people visit the doctor, with estimates showing that it affects up to 80% of adults at some point. It could be muscle-related pain, nerve-related, or disc-related pain.

Whatever the cause is, there is no denying that back pain is debilitating, especially when it moves from acute, sub-acute, recurrent, to chronic.

While there are many causes of back pain, including poor posture, sedentary lifestyles, injury, and aging, one thing is

---

[1] https://www.ncbi.nlm.nih.gov/pmc/articles/PMC1496956/

clear: a healthy spine is crucial for overall health and well-being.

But what exactly is a healthy spine, and why is it so important?

Your spine is a complex structure made up of bones, muscles, nerves, and other tissues that work together to support your body and allow you to move.

When your spine is healthy, it can withstand daily life stresses and help prevent injury and pain. But when it's not, problems can arise, including back pain, sciatica, and even more serious conditions like herniated discs.

So how can you maintain a healthy spine and prevent these issues? That's where anabolism comes in.

Anabolism is the process your body uses to build and repair tissues, including those in your spine. By optimizing your metabolism and providing your body with the right nutrients, you can support spine tissue regeneration and keep your spine healthy and strong.

This book will teach you different strategies to promote a healthy spine and prevent or cope with back pain and sciatica.

More precisely, you will discover:

- The type of water that is healthy for your spine and why.

- The power of eating vegetables in promoting the health of your spine.

- The kind of diet you ought to adopt for a healthy spine.

- How walking is better than running for your spine.

- The type of walking you should be doing for a stronger spine.

- The power of rest in promoting anabolism for a healthy spine.

- And so much more.

Let's dive into the first chapter, where we will learn about hydration and the kind of water you should drink for a healthy and strong spine.

About The Author

Dr. Edwin Roll currently runs a clinic specializing in treating sciatica pain. He has spent many years providing rehabilitation and psychological support to individuals suffering from chronic neurological conditions such as Parkinson's disease, multiple sclerosis, polyneuropathy, and fibromyalgia.

Since 2009, he has been the director of a vocational training center for physicians, physiotherapists, massage therapists, and nurses in the fundamentals of manual therapy for the musculoskeletal system. He values the use of evidence-based scientific knowledge and employs both academic theory and clinical methods in his practice, including the Cyriax Orthopaedic Medicine method, manual medicine methods such as osteopathy and soft chiropractic, and the Ackermann method.

Dr. Roll's qualifications include a degree in physiotherapy, a master's in movement rehabilitation and therapeutic pedagogy, chiropractic certification, certification as a visceral osteopath, a master's in public health, a psychotraumatology degree, an Executive MBA, and a Doctorate in Public Health.

Table of Content

Chapter 1: Proper Hydration for a Healthy Spine

Did you know proper hydration can be crucial in maintaining a healthy spine? That's right!

Water is essential for overall health and the health of your spine. What's more, boiled water is recommended instead of mineral water!

If you are curious about how this chapter will show you how water is useful for your spine's health and how boiled water is better, we shall explore the importance of proper hydration for a healthy spine.

How Does the Water You Drink Affect Your Spine?

The water we drink affects our spine in the following ways:

Hydration improves disc health

Research[2] shows that the discs between your vertebrae are responsible for cushioning your spine and absorbing the impact and pressure that your spine undergoes during daily activities.

---

[2] https://www.ncbi.nlm.nih.gov/pmc/articles/PMC6356370/

The discs have main components: the outer annulus fibrosus and the inner nucleus pulposus. The annulus fibrosus is a tough outer layer that encases the nucleus pulposus, a gel-like substance that gives the disc its shock-absorbing properties.

(A)

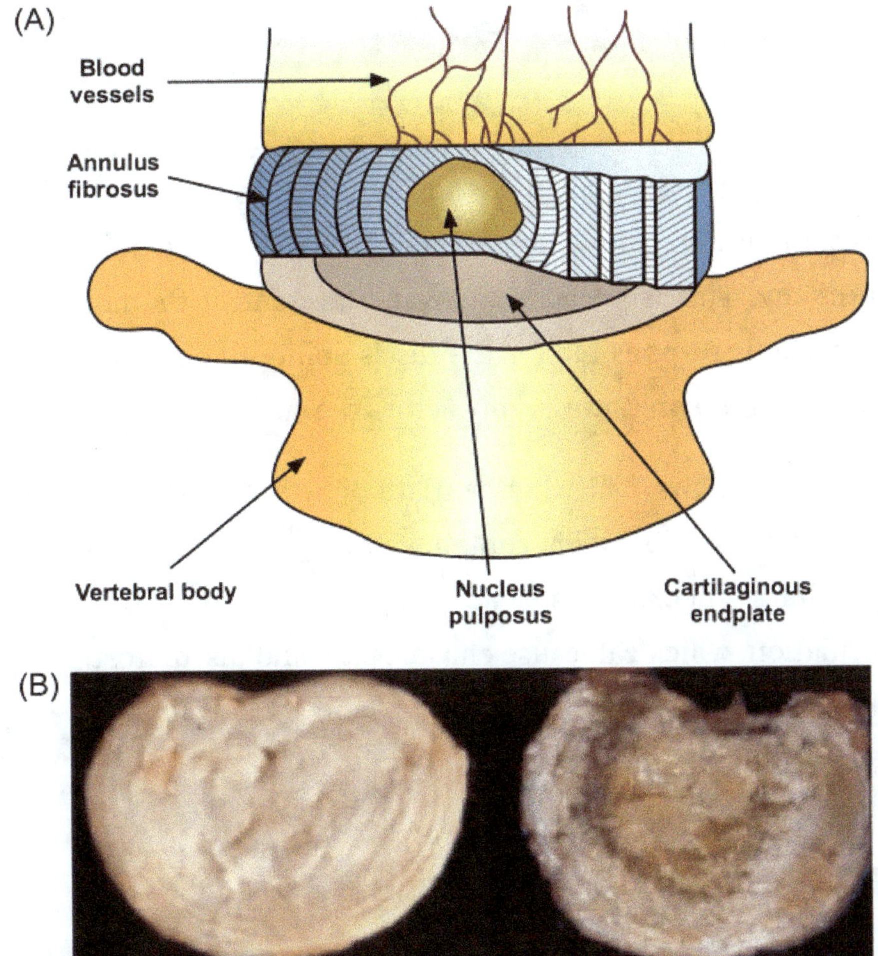

(B)

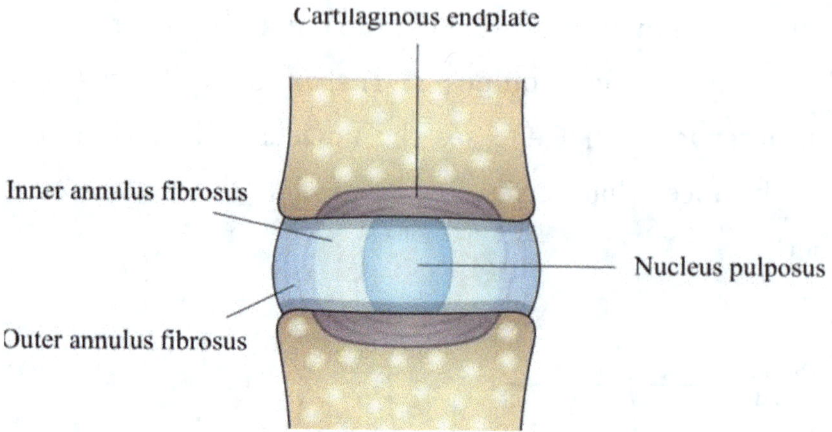

Research[3] shows that the nucleus pulposus requires a constant water supply to maintain its shape and function optimally. This is because the water content of the nucleus pulposus is responsible for the disc's ability to absorb shock and distribute pressure evenly across the spine.

Research[4] shows that when you are dehydrated, the nucleus pulposus loses its water content, making it less effective at absorbing shock. This leads to degeneration and disc herniation, which can cause chronic pain and discomfort.

[3] https://www.ncbi.nlm.nih.gov/pmc/articles/PMC6112070/
[4] https://www.ncbi.nlm.nih.gov/books/NBK441822/#:~:text=The%20most%20common%20cause%20of,herniation%20that%20can%20cause%20symptoms.

Scientific evidence[5] proves that drinking adequate water ensures your discs remain properly hydrated and functioning at their best.

Research[6] shows that the body maintains water content in the nucleus pulposus through a process called imbibition, which is the absorption of fluid into the disc through movement and pressure changes in the spine. When you drink enough water, your body is better able to facilitate this process, keeping your discs healthy and functional.

Water helps to maintain spinal alignment

Your spine protects the spinal cord and nerves, supports your upper body's weight, and maintains your posture and balance. The spine has a series of vertebrae connected by muscles, ligaments, and intervertebral discs. These structures work together to support your body's weight and allow movement.

Research[7] shows that when you are dehydrated, the water content in your muscles and ligaments decreases, making them less flexible and more prone to tension and stiffness. This can affect your spinal alignment and cause postural imbalances that can lead to chronic pain and discomfort.

---

[5] https://www.ncbi.nlm.nih.gov/pmc/articles/PMC2908954/
[6] https://www.ncbi.nlm.nih.gov/pmc/articles/PMC6112070/
[7] https://www.ncbi.nlm.nih.gov/pmc/articles/PMC6723611/

For example, research[8] shows that if the muscles in your back and neck become tight and inflexible, it can cause your spine to curve or twist, leading to spinal misalignment.

Research[9] shows that drinking enough water helps maintain spinal alignment by keeping your muscles and ligaments hydrated and flexible.

Additional research[10] has also shown that when your muscles and ligaments remain properly hydrated, they can better support your spine and maintain its natural curvature. This reduces the risk of postural imbalances and spinal misalignment, which can cause pain and discomfort.

Proper hydration promotes nutrient delivery

Water is a vital component of the body's transport system; it plays a crucial role in delivering nutrients to the cells, tissues, and organs.

Research[11] shows that nutrients such as calcium, magnesium, and vitamin D are essential for maintaining strong bones and healthy discs in the spine. Calcium and magnesium are particularly important for bone health as they provide the

---

[8] https://www.webmd.com/back-pain/causes-scoliosis
[9] https://www.cdc.gov/healthyweight/healthy_eating/water-and-healthier-drinks.html
[10] https://www.ncbi.nlm.nih.gov/pmc/articles/PMC6166197/
[11] https://www.ncbi.nlm.nih.gov/pmc/articles/PMC3330619/

structural support necessary for maintaining bone density and strength.

Research[12] shows that when you are dehydrated, your body struggles to transport nutrients to the spine, leading to a deficiency of essential nutrients. This can cause several degenerative conditions, such as osteoporosis, a condition known to weaken bones and make them more prone to fractures.

Research[13] shows that osteoporosis is particularly common in postmenopausal women who experience decreased estrogen production— estrogen is essential for maintaining bone density.

Research[14] shows proper hydration is critical for promoting nutrient delivery to the spine, ensuring that essential nutrients reach the bones and spinal discs. Water facilitates the transport of nutrients through the bloodstream, delivering them to the cells in the spine that require them.

Research[15] proves that adequate hydration ensures the cells in the spine receive the necessary nutrients, promoting

[12] https://www.ncbi.nlm.nih.gov/pmc/articles/PMC2908954/
[13] https://www.ncbi.nlm.nih.gov/pmc/articles/PMC5643776/
[14] https://www.ncbi.nlm.nih.gov/pmc/articles/PMC6112070/
[15] https://www.ncbi.nlm.nih.gov/pmc/articles/PMC8746518/

healthy bone density and reducing the risk of degenerative conditions such as osteoporosis and osteoarthritis.

In addition to promoting nutrient delivery, water helps remove waste products from the body, including those that can accumulate in the spine and contribute to degenerative conditions.

Scientific evidence[16] shows that proper hydration ensures that waste products are flushed out of the body, reducing the risk of inflammation and tissue damage in the spine.

Water helps reduce inflammation

Inflammation is the body's natural response to injury, infection, or irritation. It is a protective mechanism that helps remove damaged tissue and initiate healing.

However, research[17] shows that when inflammation becomes chronic, it can cause damage to the spinal cord and nerves, leading to chronic pain and discomfort.

Research[18] shows that drinking enough water effectively reduces inflammation in the body, including inflammation in the spine. Water helps flush out toxins from the body, which

---

[16] https://www.ncbi.nlm.nih.gov/pmc/articles/PMC2908954/
[17] https://www.ncbi.nlm.nih.gov/pmc/articles/PMC3155807/
[18] https://www.health.harvard.edu/staying-healthy/how-much-water-should-you-drink

can trigger an inflammatory response. These toxins can accumulate in the joints and spine tissues, causing inflammation and tissue damage.

Water also promotes healthy circulation, which is essential for reducing inflammation in the body. When dehydrated, your blood becomes thicker and more viscous, making it more difficult to circulate throughout the body. This can cause inflammation in the spine and other parts, leading to chronic pain and discomfort. Drinking enough water helps thin the blood, promoting healthy circulation and reducing the risk of inflammation.

Another way water can help reduce inflammation is by keeping your joints lubricated. The joints in the spine rely on a lubricating fluid called synovial fluid to reduce friction and prevent damage.

When dehydrated, your body struggles to produce enough synovial fluid, increasing the risk of inflammation and tissue damage in the spine. Drinking enough water helps keep your joints lubricated, reducing the risk of inflammation and tissue damage.

Water helps regulate body temperature

The human body has a design mechanism that helps regulate its internal temperature within a narrow range, around 98.6°F (37°C), regardless of the external temperature. The spinal cord and nerves are particularly sensitive to temperature changes, and excess heat can damage these delicate tissues.

The muscles and tissues surrounding your spine generate heat as they work to support your body and maintain your posture. Research[19] shows that ineffective heat dissipation can cause heat to accumulate in the spine, increasing the risk of damage to the spinal cord and nerves. Drinking enough water helps regulate your body temperature and prevent overheating.

Water helps regulate body temperature by facilitating sweat production. When you are dehydrated, your body struggles to produce enough sweat, which is essential for cooling the body. As a result, your body temperature can rise, increasing the risk of overheating and spinal cord and nerve damage. Drinking enough water helps keep your body hydrated, which promotes healthy sweat production and effective heat dissipation.

---

[19] https://www.ncbi.nlm.nih.gov/pmc/articles/PMC7518736/

Moreover, water is an essential component of blood. It helps regulate body temperature by transferring heat from the body's core to the skin, where the body can dissipate it through sweating.

When dehydrated, your blood becomes thicker and more viscous, making it more difficult to transfer heat effectively. Drinking enough water helps keep your blood thin and flowing smoothly, promoting effective heat transfer and keeping your spine and surrounding tissues cool.

Clearly, hydration is vital to maintaining a healthy spine. However, how many glasses of water are enough in a day?

Well, there really is no specific number of glasses of water you need to drink daily to maintain a healthy spine. Different factors come into play when thinking about how much water you should drink. These include your body weight, level of physical activity, and the climate you live in.

However, as a general guideline, research[20] recommends that as a man, you should aim to drink about 3.7 liters of water in a day, and as a woman, you should aim to drink about 2.7 liters of water in a day.

---

[20] https://www.forbes.com/health/body/how-much-water-you-should-drink-per-day/#:~:text=The%20Institute%20of%20Medicine%20of,fluid%20orather%20than%20plain%20water.

Please note that this includes water from all sources, such as beverages and food. This is the recommended daily intake for overall hydration and health, not just for spine health.

Additionally, and as mentioned, boiled water is the best water to drink:

Why Boiled Water is Better

Boiled water is a fundamental necessity for survival and a wise choice for maintaining good health.

Boiling water purifies it in a way that eliminates harmful bacteria, viruses, and other present contaminants. This makes boiled water safe and suitable for consumption, reducing the risk of waterborne illnesses and promoting overall well-being.

Boiled water is recommended for the health of your spine, as opposed to mineral water, due to the following reasons:

Water as a Substrate

Water plays a crucial role in the biochemical processes of the body, including those related to the health of your spine. It provides the environment in which these processes occur and directly participates in many of them as a reacting agent. By consuming boiled water, which is closest to the chemical formula of water (H2O) without additional minerals, you provide a pure substrate for these processes to take place.

Solvent

Water is the most important solvent in your body, capable of dissolving various nutrients, hormones, enzymes, and other essential substances. This property of water enables their transport and facilitates necessary chemical reactions. By consuming boiled water, you ensure that the water you intake is in its purest form without any added minerals.

Boiled water, devoid of minerals, serves as an effective solvent within your body. It helps in dissolving and transporting important substances that are required for the health and proper functioning of your spine. By avoiding mineral water, which contains additional minerals, you reduce the risk of introducing unwanted substances that may interfere with these processes.

Homeostasis

Water plays a vital role in maintaining fluid balance within your body, which is crucial for various functions, including the regulation of body temperature, maintenance of blood pressure, and the transport of nutrients and waste products. Boiled water, by eliminating most minerals and potential contaminants, provides a pure and balanced medium for these homeostatic processes to occur optimally.

Your spine's health relies on maintaining proper fluid balance, ensuring the delivery of nutrients and removal of waste products. By consuming boiled water, you help maintain the necessary fluid balance, allowing your spine to function optimally and ensuring the health of its discs. The absence of additional minerals in boiled water reduces the risk of potential imbalances that may affect your spine's homeostatic mechanisms.

As you would guess, boiled water is recommended for the health of your spine because it provides a pure substrate, acts as an effective solvent, and supports homeostasis. By consuming boiled water, you create an environment that promotes the efficient functioning of your spine and minimizes the introduction of additional components that may interfere with its health. Mineral water, on the other hand, primarily serves the purpose of mineralization, which may not be as directly beneficial for the specific needs of your spine.

That said, let's look at what your diet should look like if you want to maintain optimum spine health.

Chapter 2: The Right Diet for a Healthy Spine

Did you know that your diet can play a crucial role in the health of your spine? Well, now you know. Making the right food choices can help you reduce pain, prevent injuries, and improve your overall quality of life.

This chapter will explore the foods and nutrients considered essential for a healthy spine and the ones to avoid to fuel your body for optimal spinal health!

The Power of Cooked Vegetables in Boosting Your Spine Health

Vegetables are a huge part of a healthy diet, and they are great for spine health for the following reasons:

Vegetables are rich in vitamins and minerals

Vitamins and minerals play a crucial role in maintaining spine health. Calcium and magnesium are two minerals considered particularly important for the bones in the spine.

These minerals work together to build strong, healthy bones resistant to fractures and degeneration. Research[21] shows

---

[21] https://www.ncbi.nlm.nih.gov/pmc/articles/PMC3775240/

that without adequate calcium and magnesium intake, the bones in the spine can become weak and brittle, increasing the risk of fractures and other spine-related conditions.

Vitamin C has been proven by research to be another nutrient that is important for spine health. Research[22] shows that Vitamin C has been proven by research to be vital in producing collagen, a protein found in the body's connective tissues, including spinal discs. Collagen helps maintain the discs' strength and elasticity, which are essential for absorbing shock and preventing injury to the spine.

Research[23] shows that vitamin D is also important for spine health. It helps the body absorb calcium, which promotes strong bones. Low vitamin D levels are a known cause of an increased risk of osteoporosis, a condition that weakens the bones and can lead to fractures in the spine.

Incorporating a variety of vegetables into your diet can help ensure you get the vitamins and minerals your spine needs to stay healthy.

Leafy green vegetables such as spinach and kale are particularly good sources of calcium and magnesium; citrus

---

[22] https://www.ncbi.nlm.nih.gov/pmc/articles/PMC6204628/
[23] https://www.ncbi.nlm.nih.gov/pmc/articles/PMC2621390/

fruits and bell peppers are high in vitamin C. Mushrooms and fatty fish such as salmon are good sources of vitamin D.

Eating a balanced diet with plenty of vegetables can help keep your spine healthy and strong for years to come.

Vegetables contain antioxidants

Antioxidants are compounds found in many fruits and vegetables; they help protect the body against the damaging effects of free radicals. Free radicals are unstable molecules that can damage cells, including those in the spine. This damage can contribute to spinal degeneration, leading to herniated discs, spinal stenosis, osteoarthritis, and many other conditions.

Research[24] shows that eating a diet high in antioxidants, including vegetables, can help neutralize free radicals and protect the cells in the spine from damage.

Vegetables such as broccoli, carrots, and sweet potatoes are particularly good sources of antioxidants, including vitamin C and beta-carotene. These antioxidants can help reduce spine inflammation, a known common contributor to back pain.

---

[24] https://www.nccih.nih.gov/health/antioxidants-in-depth

In addition to vitamin C and beta-carotene, vegetables have many other antioxidants, including quercetin, lutein, and zeaxanthin. These antioxidants have a research-proven[25] ability to have anti-inflammatory and immune-boosting properties, which can help protect the spine against a range of conditions.

It's important to note that the antioxidants in vegetables are most effective when consumed in their natural form rather than in supplement form. Eating a varied diet that includes a range of colorful vegetables can help ensure you get a range of antioxidants that support the health of your spine and overall health.

Vegetables are low in calories

Maintaining a healthy weight is important for overall health, particularly the spine's health. Research[26] shows that being overweight or obese can put extra stress on the spine and increase the risk of developing spine-related conditions such as herniated discs, spinal stenosis, and osteoarthritis.

Vegetables are an excellent choice for those looking to maintain a healthy weight or lose weight because they are low in calories but high in essential nutrients.

---

[25] https://www.ncbi.nlm.nih.gov/pmc/articles/PMC7575721/
[26] https://www.ncbi.nlm.nih.gov/pmc/articles/PMC5334737/

For example, research[27] shows that one cup of cooked broccoli contains just 55 calories but provides a significant amount of vitamin C, K, and fiber. Similarly, one medium-sized carrot contains just 25 calories but is rich in vitamins A, K, and fiber.

In addition to being low in calories, vegetables are also high in fiber. Fiber helps keep you feeling full, which can prevent overeating and unhealthy snacking. By incorporating more vegetables into your diet, you can reduce your calorie intake while ensuring you get the nutrients your body needs to function properly.

Vegetables are high in fiber

Fiber is a crucial nutrient that helps maintain a healthy digestive system. Vegetables are an excellent source of dietary fiber, which can help keep the digestive system running smoothly. When it comes to spine health, a healthy digestive system is also essential.

Research[28] shows that constipation is a common issue that can strain the lower back and contribute to back pain.

[27] https://www.scirp.org/html/4-2700478_23384.htm
[28] https://www.medicalnewstoday.com/articles/325663

Fortunately, scientific evidence[29] proves that eating a diet high in fiber, including plenty of vegetables can help prevent constipation and promote regular bowel movements.

Keeping the digestive system at optimal functionality reduces the risk of developing spine-related conditions caused by straining during bowel movements.

Vegetables are anti-inflammatory

Inflammation is the body's natural process in response to injury or infection. However, research[30] shows that when inflammation becomes chronic, it can contribute to various health issues, including back pain and other spine-related conditions. Vegetables are a great source of anti-inflammatory compounds that can help to reduce inflammation in the body.

One group of anti-inflammatory compounds found in vegetables is flavonoids. Flavonoids are a type of phytonutrient research[31] has proven to have anti-inflammatory properties.

[29]https://www.ncbi.nlm.nih.gov/pmc/articles/PMC7589116/
[30] https://www.ncbi.nlm.nih.gov/pmc/articles/PMC5744892/
[31]https://www.ncbi.nlm.nih.gov/pmc/articles/PMC5465813/

Vegetables like kale, broccoli, and Brussels sprouts are particularly high in flavonoids. These compounds can help reduce inflammation in the body and protect the spine from damage caused by chronic inflammation.

Another group of anti-inflammatory compounds found in vegetables is carotenoids. Carotenoids are another type of phytonutrient that research[32] has proven to have anti-inflammatory properties.

Vegetables such as carrots, sweet potatoes, and spinach are particularly high in carotenoids. These compounds can help reduce inflammation in the body and protect the spine from damage caused by chronic inflammation.

In addition to flavonoids and carotenoids, vegetables are a great source of other anti-inflammatory nutrients such as vitamins C, E, and beta-carotene. These nutrients work together to reduce inflammation and promote overall health and well-being.

Vegetables are low in sugar

Excess sugar consumption is a well-known cause of various health problems, including inflammation and chronic pain.

---

[32]https://www.mdpi.com/2076-3921/12/3/676#:~:text=A%20growing%20body%20of%20evidence,the%20risk%20of%20developing%20depression.

Consuming too much sugar can cause inflammation in the body and trigger the release of pro-inflammatory compounds that can contribute to chronic conditions like back pain.

Vegetables are naturally low in sugar and provide a healthy alternative to sugary foods and beverages. By incorporating more vegetables into your diet, you can help reduce your overall sugar intake and maintain a healthy balance in your diet. This is particularly important for spine health because excess sugar consumption can increase the risk of developing back pain.

Excess sugar consumption has been scientifically linked[33] to numerous negative health effects, including an increased risk of developing back pain. Studies[34] have shown that consuming high levels of sugar can lead to chronic inflammation, which can contribute to a range of health problems, including back pain.

Consuming large amounts of sugar can cause our bodies to produce higher levels of inflammatory cytokines, which are proteins released by the immune system in response to inflammation. These cytokines can cause inflammation in the

---

[33] https://www.ncbi.nlm.nih.gov/pmc/articles/PMC5133084/#:~:text=Con sumption%20of%20added%20sugars%20has,decline%20and%20even%20some%20cancers.
[34] https://www.ncbi.nlm.nih.gov/pmc/articles/PMC9471313/

muscles and joints of the back, leading to pain and discomfort.

Vegetables contain phytonutrients

Phytonutrients are naturally occurring compounds found in plants. Research[35] has shown that these compounds have numerous health benefits, including anti-inflammatory and antioxidant properties. These compounds can help reduce inflammation in the body and protect against oxidative stress that can contribute to a range of health problems, including spine-related conditions.

Vegetables are a great source of phytonutrients, and by eating a variety of colorful vegetables, you can ensure you get a range of these important compounds.

For example, cruciferous vegetables such as broccoli and kale are rich in sulforaphane, a phytonutrient that research[36] has proven to have anti-inflammatory and anti-cancer properties.

---

[35] https://www.ncbi.nlm.nih.gov/pmc/articles/PMC9102588/

[36] https://www.healthline.com/nutrition/sulforaphane#:~:text=Sulforaphane%20is%20a%20natural%20plant,improved%20heart%20health%20and%20digestion.

Research[37] has also shown that Carotenoids, another group of phytonutrients found in vegetables such as carrots and sweet potatoes, have antioxidant properties that may help reduce spinal inflammation.

Vegetables are a good source of hydration

As discussed in the first chapter, water plays a crucial role in promoting the health of your spine. Research[38] shows that vegetables are a great source of hydration, as many veggies are high in water content.

For example, cucumbers are over 95% water, while celery is over 95% water. Other vegetables, such as lettuce, tomatoes, and zucchini, are also high in water content and can help keep you hydrated throughout the day.

In addition to helping to maintain spinal disc health, staying hydrated can also help reduce inflammation and improve the overall health and function of the body.

Including a variety of hydrating vegetables in your diet can help support a healthy spine and overall well-being.

---

[37] https://www.ncbi.nlm.nih.gov/pmc/articles/PMC9102588/
[38] https://www.bupa.co.uk/newsroom/ourviews/ten-water-rich-foods-hydration#:~:text=Cucumbers%20are%20made%20up%20of,to%20make%20a%20refreshing%20drink.

Why Cook Your Vegetables?

Cooked vegetables are better than raw vegetables in promoting the health of your spine due to the following reasons:

Enhanced Nutrient Absorption

Cooking vegetables can facilitate the digestion and absorption of certain nutrients present in them. When vegetables are cooked, the cellular structures break down, making it easier for your body to access and absorb the nutrients they contain. This enhanced nutrient absorption can be particularly beneficial for the health of your spine.

By cooking vegetables, you increase the availability and accessibility of nutrients that are essential for the health of your spine. The breakdown of cellular structures during cooking allows your body to digest and absorb these nutrients more effectively, ensuring that they reach the necessary areas, such as the spinal discs, where they are needed for optimal functioning.

Increased Bioavailability of Phytonutrients

Cooking certain vegetables can significantly increase the bioavailability of specific phytonutrients that have been associated with various health benefits. For example, research[39] shows that when tomatoes are cooked, the bioavailability of lycopene, an antioxidant known for its potential protective effects on spinal health, increases.

Cooking tomatoes helps release and enhance the bioavailability of lycopene, making it easier for your body to absorb and utilize this beneficial antioxidant. By consuming cooked tomatoes, you provide your spine with a higher concentration of lycopene, potentially promoting its health.

Improved Beta-Carotene Absorption

Certain vegetables, such as carrots, contain beta-carotene, a precursor to vitamin A and an essential nutrient for spine health. Research[40] shows that cooking carrots can increase the bioavailability of beta-carotene, allowing your body to absorb and utilize it more efficiently.

Beta-carotene plays a vital role in maintaining the health of your spine due to its conversion into vitamin A, which is essential for bone growth and maintenance. Cooking carrots breaks down the cell walls, making the beta-carotene more accessible and easier to absorb. By consuming cooked carrots, you enhance the absorption and utilization of beta-carotene, promoting the health of your spine.

---

[39] https://www.ncbi.nlm.nih.gov/pmc/articles/PMC7464847/
[40] https://pubmed.ncbi.nlm.nih.gov/14673607/

Easier Digestion

Cooking vegetables can make them easier to digest compared to consuming them raw. The process of cooking softens the fiber in vegetables, making them more gentle on your digestive system.

Some raw vegetables, particularly those with high fiber content, can be challenging for your digestive system to break down effectively. Cooking vegetables softens their fiber, making them easier to digest. This can be beneficial for your overall digestive health, ensuring that the nutrients from the cooked vegetables are absorbed and utilized optimally, including those that contribute to the health of your spine.

Apart from vegetables, what else should you consume for a healthy spine? Let's find out in the next chapter.

Chapter 3: Eating Like a Small Child for a Healthy Spine

The previous chapter discussed why vegetables are essential in maintaining spine health. However, you cannot live on vegetables alone. That said, what else should you eat?

Well, what if I told you that you could find the key to a healthy spine in the eating habits of small children? As strange as it may sound, it's true because children's diets are rich in nutrients essential for spinal health and development.

This chapter will explore the science behind this idea and outline practical tips to help you eat like a small child to improve your spinal health and overall well-being.

So, get ready to embrace your inner child and learn how to nourish your spine like never before!

What Should Your Diet Look Like?

You're probably wondering what eating like a small child entails and how it relates to the health of your spine.

Well, without beating around the bush, let's look at the different foods you should eat to boost your spine health. Mostly, we focus on giving our kids these foods without knowing that they could benefit us as well:

Dairy products

Research[41] shows that calcium is the main building block for bones and is crucial for maintaining the health and strength of the spine.

Dairy products are one of the best sources of calcium and are readily available in most households. Cheese, yogurt, and milk are delicious and great sources of calcium, making them ideal for supporting bone and spine health.

In addition to calcium, research[42] shows that dairy products are also rich in vitamin D, which is essential for the absorption and utilization of calcium in the body. Vitamin D helps regulate calcium and phosphorus levels in the blood, and vitamin D deficiency can result in weakened bones, high risks of fractures, and muscle weakness.

Consuming dairy products regularly, in combination with other vitamin D sources, such as sunlight exposure, can help support spine health and minimize the chances of spinal conditions like osteoporosis.

---

[41] https://www.ncbi.nlm.nih.gov/pmc/articles/PMC6316542/
[42] https://www.ncbi.nlm.nih.gov/pmc/articles/PMC7353177/

Fatty fish

Fatty fish like salmon, sardines, and tuna are delicious and packed with health-boosting nutrients.

Research[43] shows that one of the key nutrients found in these fish is omega-3 fatty acids which play an important role in maintaining spine health. Omega-3 can aid in reducing inflammation in the spine, thereby alleviating pain and stiffness.

Inflammation is the way your body responds to infections. However, when you're too chronically inflamed, you can start suffering from various spinal conditions like arthritis and degenerative disc disease. Consuming fatty fish regularly can help manage inflammation and minimize the chances of these conditions.

Furthermore, research[44] shows that omega-3 fatty acids may help improve blood flow to the spine and minimize the chances of blood clots. Blood clots can cause serious health problems and may lead to life-altering conditions like stroke or heart attack.

Fatty fish can help improve circulation and prevent blood clots from forming, which can be especially beneficial for

---

[43] https://www.ncbi.nlm.nih.gov/pmc/articles/PMC3262608/
[44] https://www.ncbi.nlm.nih.gov/pmc/articles/PMC4153275/

those with spinal cord injuries or conditions that affect blood flow to the spine.

Overall, incorporating fatty fish into your diet can help support spine health and minimize the chnces of of spinal conditions caused by inflammation and poor circulation.

Nuts and seeds

Nuts and seeds are a delicious and easy way to incorporate magnesium into your diet, an essential mineral that vitally supports bone and spine health.

Research[45] shows that almonds, chia seeds, and pumpkin seeds are excellent sources of magnesium, which the body needs to form strong bones and healthy nerve function.

Magnesium also plays a crucial role in regulating muscle contractions, including those of the muscles that support the spine. Muscle cramps and spasms can occur without adequate magnesium, exacerbating spinal pain.

Studies[46] have shown that magnesium may also have a role in reducing inflammation in the body, which can contribute to spinal conditions like osteoarthritis and rheumatoid arthritis.

---

[45] https://ods.od.nih.gov/factsheets/Magnesium-HealthProfessional/
[46] https://www.ncbi.nlm.nih.gov/pmc/articles/PMC7654130/

Incorporating nuts and seeds into your diet can be an easy way to increase your magnesium intake and support spine health. It's important to note that consuming too much magnesium can have adverse effects, so it's essential to consume these foods in moderation and follow recommended daily intake guidelines.

Leafy greens

Leafy greens are particularly beneficial for spine health as they contain vitamin K, an essential nutrient for strong bones, including those in the spine.

Research[47] shows that vitamin K helps regulate calcium absorption and deposition in the bones, making them stronger and less prone to fractures. Vitamin K also plays a role in synthesizing osteocalcin, a protein necessary for bone mineralization. This means regularly consuming leafy greens can help maintain bone density and prevent osteoporosis, a condition in which bones become weak and brittle, increasing the risk of fractures and spinal deformities.

In addition to vitamin K, leafy greens contain other important nutrients like vitamin A, vitamin C, and folate, which support overall health and are essential for the proper functioning of the body.

---

[47] https://www.ncbi.nlm.nih.gov/pmc/articles/PMC7760385/

Vitamin A, for example, is important for the growth and repair of tissues, including those in the spine. In contrast, scientific research has proven that Vitamin C is an antioxidant that helps protect cells from free radical damage. Folate, on the other hand, is very crucial for the production of red blood cells and helps prevent congenital disabilities.

Regularly consuming leafy greens can also help reduce inflammation, which is beneficial for preventing conditions like osteoarthritis and degenerative disc disease, which can cause spinal pain and stiffness.

Berries

Berries are delicious and incredibly nutritious, making them an excellent addition to your diet to support spine health. Strawberries, blueberries, and raspberries are all packed with antioxidants that protect the body from the harmful effects of free radicals.

Free radicals are unstable molecules that can damage cells and contribute to inflammation and oxidative stress, harming the spinal cord and increasing the risk of spinal conditions like herniated discs.

Luckily, research[48] has proven that regularly consuming berries can help fight off free radicals and protect the spine from damage.

In addition to antioxidants, berries are rich in vitamin C, a vital nutrient known to support collagen production. Collagen is a protein that makes up the cartilage that cushions the spine and other joints.

Research[49] shows that Vitamin C is essential for collagen synthesis, and a deficiency in this vitamin can lead to weakened cartilage and an increased risk of spinal conditions like degenerative disc disease.

Consuming berries regularly as part of a balanced diet can help ensure your body has adequate vitamin C to support the health of the spine's cushioning cartilage and minimize the chances of spinal conditions.

Whole grains

Incorporating whole grains into your diet is an easy and delicious way to support spine health. Whole wheat bread, quinoa, and brown rice are all excellent sources of fiber, which plays a crucial role in regulating bowel movements and reducing inflammation throughout the body.

[48] https://www.healthline.com/nutrition/11-reasons-to-eat-berries
[49] https://www.ncbi.nlm.nih.gov/pmc/articles/PMC3783921/

Chronic inflammation can lead to tissue damage in the spine and contribute to conditions like osteoporosis and spinal stenosis. Research[50] shows that eating whole grains can help regulate inflammation levels in the human body, reducing the risk of spinal conditions.

In addition to fiber, whole grains are also rich in B vitamins, which crucially support healthy nerve function. The spine has many nerves that transmit signals to and from the brain, enabling movement and sensation throughout the body.

Scientific studies[51] have shown that B vitamins help support the health of these nerves, ensuring that they function correctly and reducing the risk of nerve-related spinal conditions like sciatica.

Incorporating whole grains like whole wheat bread, quinoa, and brown rice into your diet can give your body the essential nutrients needed to maintain a healthy spine and minimize the chances of spinal conditions.

---

[50] https://www.ncbi.nlm.nih.gov/pmc/articles/PMC6221555/
[51] https://www.ncbi.nlm.nih.gov/pmc/articles/PMC8294980/

Lean protein

Incorporating lean protein into your diet can have significant benefits for spine health.

Lean protein sources such as chicken, lean beef, and turkey are essential for building and repairing tissues in the body, including the muscles that support the spine. Muscles play a crucial role in supporting the spine and maintaining good posture.

Research[52] shows that consuming adequate amounts of lean protein can help ensure these muscles are strong and capable of effectively supporting the spine.

Additionally, protein is essential for healthy bone growth and maintenance. Adequate protein intake can help maintain bone density and minimize the chances of health conditions like osteoporosis, weakening the spine and increasing the risk of fractures.

In addition to their muscle-building and bone-strengthening properties, lean protein sources are rich in essential vitamins and minerals. Chicken, turkey, and lean beef are excellent sources of essential B vitamins that support nerve function and iron, which helps transport oxygen to tissues throughout

---

[52] https://www.ncbi.nlm.nih.gov/pmc/articles/PMC4180248/

the body, including the spine. These foods are also rich in zinc, which plays a role in bone formation and maintenance.

Incorporating lean protein sources into your diet can give your body the essential nutrients it needs to support spine health and overall health.

Citrus fruits

Citrus fruits are a great addition to any diet, especially for those looking to support spine health. These fruits, including lemons, oranges, and grapefruits, are rich in vitamin C, an essential nutrient that research[53] has shown is important for collagen production. Collagen is the protein that makes up the cartilage in the spine and other joints, and a lack of vitamin C can lead to weakened cartilage and increased spinal pain.

Research[54] also shows that vitamin C plays a crucial role in the formation, maintenance, and repair of connective tissues throughout the body, including the cartilage in the spine.

Without adequate vitamin C, the body may not be able to produce enough collagen to keep the cartilage healthy and strong. This can lead to health conditions like osteoarthritis,

---

[53] https://www.hsph.harvard.edu/nutritionsource/vitamin-c/
[54] https://www.ncbi.nlm.nih.gov/pmc/articles/PMC4833003/

a degenerative joint disease that can cause pain and stiffness in the spine and other joints.

Incorporating citrus fruits into your diet can ensure your body gets the vitamin C it needs to support healthy cartilage and minimize the chances of spinal pain and degeneration.

In addition to supporting the production of collagen, Vitamin C has been proven by research to be a powerful antioxidant that helps protect the body from damage caused by free radicals. Research[55] shows that free radicals can contribute to inflammation and oxidative stress that can damage the spinal cord and increase the risk of spinal conditions like herniated discs.

Regularly consuming citrus fruits can help keep free radicals at bay and protect the spine from damage. So, adding citrus fruits to your diet can support spine health and boost overall health and well-being.

Red and orange vegetables

Carotenoids are pigments found in red and orange vegetables and are popular for their anti-inflammatory properties. In addition to protecting the spine from damage caused by free

---

[55] https://www.ncbi.nlm.nih.gov/pmc/articles/PMC9315394/

radicals, research[56] shows that carotenoids may also help reduce inflammation in the body.

Chronic inflammation can damage the spine and contribute to conditions like osteoporosis and spinal stenosis, so including red and orange vegetables in your diet can be a great way to support spinal health.

Furthermore, these vegetables are also rich in vitamin A, which is important for maintaining healthy vision, skin, and immune function.

Incorporating red and orange vegetables into your meals can be simple and delicious. Adding sliced peppers to salads or stir-fries, roasting sweet potatoes for a side dish, or snacking on baby carrots with hummus are all easy ways to increase your intake of these nutrient-dense foods.

By including these colorful vegetables in your diet, you can provide your body with the antioxidants and nutrients it needs to maintain a healthy spine and overall well-being.

---

[56] https://www.ncbi.nlm.nih.gov/pmc/articles/PMC8531419/

Beans and legumes

Beans and legumes are a great addition to any diet because they are nutrient-dense and have numerous health benefits. Research[57] shows that beans and legumes are particularly beneficial for spine health because of their high fiber content, which can help regulate bowel movements and reduce inflammation in the body.

Inflammation is a major contributor to spinal conditions like osteoporosis and degenerative disc disease, so incorporating beans and legumes into your diet can help reduce your risk of developing these conditions.

Furthermore, research[58] proves that beans and legumes are a great source of plant-based protein, which is essential for building and repairing tissues in the body, including the muscles that support the spine.

They are also rich in minerals like magnesium and potassium, which are important for healthy nerve and muscle function. Magnesium, in particular, is important for regulating muscle contractions, including those in the muscles that support the spine. A magnesium deficiency can

[57] https://www.ncbi.nlm.nih.gov/pmc/articles/PMC7915747/
[58] https://www.ncbi.nlm.nih.gov/pmc/articles/PMC7915747/

lead to muscle cramps and spasms that can exacerbate spinal pain.

Therefore, incorporating beans and legumes into your diet can help support healthy nerve and muscle function, ultimately contributing to a healthier spine.

Eggs

Eggs are an excellent food source for spine health due to their high vitamin D content.

Research[59] shows that vitamin D is important for calcium absorption, and calcium is crucial for the development and maintenance of strong bones, including those in the spine.

Scientific evidence has linked[60] vitamin D deficiency to a higher risk of bone fractures, weak spine, osteoporosis, and other bone-related disorders. While eggs are not the only vitamin D food source, they are a convenient and affordable option for maintaining adequate levels of this essential nutrient.

---

[59] https://www.ncbi.nlm.nih.gov/pmc/articles/PMC2621390/
[60] https://www.ncbi.nlm.nih.gov/pmc/articles/PMC3591184/

In addition to vitamin D, eggs are also rich in protein, which is important for muscle growth and repair. The muscles surrounding the spine support and stabilize the spine; maintaining their strength is crucial for spine health.

Consuming adequate protein from sources like eggs can help support muscle growth and repair, especially when combined with regular exercise. Eating eggs for breakfast or incorporating them into meals throughout the day can help support spine health by providing important nutrients like vitamin D and protein.

By incorporating all these foods into your diet, you will be eating healthy, just like a small child, which will greatly boost your spine's health.

Let's now move away from diets and look at how you can boost the health of your spine through exercise.

Chapter 4: The Right Exercise for a Healthy Spine

Do you find yourself avoiding exercise altogether because of how much it strains your spine? The good news is that there is a solution!

This chapter will explore the benefits of incorporating the right exercise type into your routine to promote a healthy spine.

Specifically, we will focus on why walking is a better option than running and why using a treadmill is better than outdoor walking, especially if you have spine injuries or pain.

By the end of this chapter, you'll know to make the right exercise choices for a healthier, pain-free spine.

Why is Walking Better than Running for the Spine?

Walking is better for the spine than running because:

Lower impact on the spine

Running produces a much higher impact on the spine than walking because, with the former, the foot strikes the ground with force equivalent to 2-3 times the body weight. This repeated impact can cause micro-trauma to the spinal discs, leading to degeneration and pain.

Conversely, walking has a lower impact on the spine, reducing the risk of disc injury and damage.

Reduced risk of spinal compression

When running, the spine experiences compressive forces that can lead to spinal disc compression and nerve irritation. Conversely, walking distributes the load more evenly across the spine, reducing the risk of compression and nerve irritation.

Less muscle tension

Running can cause tension in the neck, shoulders, and back muscles, which can contribute to spine pain.

On the other hand, walking can help release muscle tension and promote relaxation, which is beneficial for spinal health.

Lower risk of injury

Running increases the risk of injury to the spine and other body parts, particularly if done excessively or with poor form. On the other hand, walking is a low-impact exercise with a lower risk of injury, making it a safer option for spine health.

Sustainable exercise routine

Unlike running, walking is a sustainable exercise routine that you can maintain for a longer duration and perform no matter your age and fitness levels. It is a simple and accessible exercise that is easy to incorporate into your daily routine, promoting consistency and long-term spine health benefits.

Walking is a safer and more sustainable exercise option for promoting a healthy and strong spine, especially if you have a history of spine injuries or pain. However, what kind of walking should you do?

Research[61] shows that treadmill walking is better than outdoor walking for spine rehabilitation.

Let's find out why.

Why is Treadmill Walking Better than Outdoor Walking for Boosting Spine Health?

Here are a few reasons why it is better to walk on a treadmill instead of outdoors when you want to strengthen or rehabilitate your spine:

---

[61] https://www.ncbi.nlm.nih.gov/pmc/articles/PMC4478607/

Controlled environment

The controlled environment of a treadmill is particularly beneficial for spine rehabilitation and strengthening because it allows you to adjust the settings to meet your specific needs and goals.

With a treadmill, you can modify your workout's incline, speed, and duration to prevent overstressing your spine. A treadmill allows you to gradually increase the intensity and duration of your workout without risking further injury or setbacks.

You can start with a slow speed and flat incline and then gradually increase both as your spine strengthens and becomes more resilient. This gradual approach to rehabilitation is essential for building endurance and preventing re-injury.

Furthermore, the controlled environment of a treadmill can be useful if you have limited access to safe outdoor walking areas or live in areas with extreme weather conditions.

Walking outdoors can be challenging or even dangerous in certain weather conditions, such as extreme heat or cold, heavy rain, or snow. A treadmill provides a safe and convenient alternative to outdoor walking, allowing you to continue your spine rehabilitation and strengthening routine regardless of the weather.

Consistent surface

The consistent surface of a treadmill is a significant advantage over outdoor walking, particularly when it comes to spine rehabilitation and strengthening.

The consistent surface of a treadmill means the ground beneath your feet does not change, providing a stable and secure base for walking. This stability is especially important for those with balance issues or those recovering from a spine injury because any sudden movements or jarring impacts could further damage the spine.

In contrast, outdoor walking poses several risks to those with spinal injuries or balance issues. Uneven surfaces, such as rocky trails or uneven sidewalks, can increase the risk of falls or twisted ankles.

Moreover, outdoor surfaces are not always predictable and are prone to different factors like weather changes. For instance, a once-dry surface can become slippery when it rains, increasing the risk of falls.

By contrast, the consistent surface of a treadmill reduces the risk of tripping, slipping, or falling, providing a safe and stable platform for walking. This allows individuals with spine injuries or balance issues to focus on their rehabilitation and strengthening routine without fearing further injury.

Furthermore, the consistent surface of a treadmill provides a more controlled environment for walking, which can be important for those undergoing spine rehabilitation or strengthening.

The treadmill's surface uses a design that absorbs shock, reducing the impact on your joints and spine, which is important for those recovering from spinal injuries or conditions. This reduces the risk of aggravating existing injuries or developing new ones and ensures that your spine can continue to strengthen safely.

Better posture

Posture is an important aspect of spine rehabilitation and strengthening. Good posture reduces the risk of further injury and helps alleviate pain and discomfort associated with spine conditions.

Treadmill walking can help improve posture by providing a stable and supportive environment for walking.

Unlike outdoor walking, where you may have to navigate uneven surfaces and obstacles, a treadmill provides a smooth and stable surface, allowing you to focus on proper posture and form.

Moreover, a treadmill has safety features such as handrails that provide additional support and can assist in maintaining proper posture while walking. The handrails can also help you maintain balance and minimize the chnces of of falls, which is especially important for anyone recovering from spine injuries or conditions.

Furthermore, a treadmill's adjustable incline and speed features can also help improve posture. Walking on an incline can engage different muscles in your back and core, promoting better posture and stability.

Additionally, the function to adjust the speed allows you to walk at a comfortable pace and maintain good form without compromising safety.

In contrast, outdoor walking can be more challenging, especially with maintaining proper posture. Uneven surfaces and obstacles can cause you to shift your weight and posture, increasing the risk of further injury.

Moreover, there are no safety features to assist in maintaining proper posture, and you may not always have access to a supportive surface to walk on.

Consistent speed

Maintaining a consistent speed is essential to spine rehabilitation and strengthening, and a treadmill has this advantage over outdoor walking.

A treadmill allows you to set a specific speed, ensuring you maintain a consistent pace throughout your workout. This is particularly important if you are recovering from spine surgery or injury because it allows you to gradually increase your activity levels and build endurance without risking further damage to your spine.

Moreover, consistent speed can also be beneficial for building endurance. By gradually increasing the treadmill's speed over time, you can challenge your body and build endurance while maintaining proper form and reducing the risk of injury.

On the other hand, outdoor walking can be unpredictable, and it can be challenging to maintain a consistent speed. Factors such as terrain, weather conditions, and traffic can all affect your speed, making it difficult to maintain a consistent pace.

This unpredictability can be a disadvantage for spine rehabilitation and strengthening, as it can be challenging to gradually increase your activity levels while maintaining proper form and reducing the risk of further injury.

Additionally, the consistent speed a treadmill provides can help with progress monitoring. By tracking your speed and distance on a treadmill, you can easily monitor your progress and adjust your routine as needed. This can be particularly beneficial for those recovering from spine surgery or injury, as it allows you to track your progress and adjust your routine as you regain strength and endurance.

Weather-independent

Treadmill walking offers the significant advantage of being weather-independent, making it an ideal option for spine rehabilitation and strengthening. This is especially important for individuals living in areas with extreme weather conditions that can make outdoor walking unsafe or challenging.

Weather conditions such as extreme heat, cold, rain, or snow can make outdoor walking uncomfortable, hazardous, or even impossible. These weather conditions can negatively impact the body, making it difficult to maintain proper form and reducing the workout's effectiveness. Additionally, for individuals recovering from spine surgery or injury, exposure to extreme weather conditions can be detrimental to their recovery process.

In contrast, a treadmill provides a comfortable and safe environment for walking regardless of the weather conditions outside. You can set the speed and incline to create the ideal workout conditions. You can also control the temperature and humidity levels to ensure a comfortable workout. This allows you to maintain proper form and minimize the chances of further injury while ensuring a safe and effective workout.

Safe and convenient

Treadmill walking is a safe and convenient exercise option you can do at any time of day and from the comfort of your home or gym. This is beneficial if you have a busy schedule or feel uncomfortable walking alone outdoors.

Overall, treadmill walking is a safe, effective, and convenient exercise option for strengthening and rehabilitating the spine. Its controlled environment, consistent surface, and reduced impact on the spine makes it a better option than outdoor walking for those with spinal injuries or conditions.

The Right Settings for a Treadmill

When using a treadmill walking to promote better spine health and strength, it's important to consider the settings that can optimize your workout and minimize the risk of spinal strain or injury.

Here are some key factors to keep in mind:

Incline

Utilizing the incline feature on a treadmill can help engage your core muscles and promote proper spinal alignment.

A slight incline, around 1-2%, mimics the natural movement of walking or running uphill and encourages a more upright posture, reducing stress on the spine.

Speed

Adjust the speed of the treadmill according to your fitness level and comfort. Gradually increase the speed to challenge yourself, but always prioritize safety and listen to your body. Maintaining a controlled and moderate pace allows for proper form and reduces the risk of excessive impact on the spine.

Duration and Intensity

Start with shorter durations and gradually increase the length of your treadmill sessions as your fitness level improves. Avoid overexertion and listen to your body's cues. Balancing the intensity of your workout with adequate rest periods allows your spine to recover and adapt to the physical demands.

Remember, it's always a good idea to consult a healthcare professional or a certified fitness trainer to determine the best settings and exercise routine that suits your needs and goals.

By paying attention to these factors and utilizing the appropriate settings, you can enhance your treadmill workouts to support better spine health and strength.

Exactly How Does Walking Boost Spine Health?

Having understood why treadmill walking is better than outdoor walking, let's look at how walking helps boost your spine health:

Encourages proper spinal alignment

Walking helps promote proper spinal alignment by reducing the pressure exerted on the spine. This can be especially beneficial for individuals who suffer from chronic back pain.

Studies[62] have shown that walking on a treadmill can significantly reduce the compressive force on the spine compared to other forms of exercise, making it a great option for individuals looking to improve their spine health.

Increases spinal flexibility

Treadmill walking may also increase spinal flexibility, thereby improving overall spine health. Walking on a treadmill helps stretch and loosen the muscles and ligaments surrounding the spine, reducing stiffness and improving mobility.

Additionally, a study[63] published in the Journal of Exercise Rehabilitation found that walking on a treadmill can significantly increase spinal flexibility in older adults.

---

[62] https://www.ncbi.nlm.nih.gov/pmc/articles/PMC4934575/
[63] https://www.ncbi.nlm.nih.gov/pmc/articles/PMC4934575/

Improves posture

Walking on a treadmill can help improve posture by strengthening the muscles that support the spine. This can be especially beneficial for individuals who spend long hours sitting at a desk or in front of a computer.

Studies[64] have shown that regular treadmill walking can improve posture and minimize the chances of developing spinal problems such as kyphosis or scoliosis.

Builds core strength

Treadmill walking is an excellent way to build core strength, which is essential for maintaining a healthy spine. Walking on a treadmill engages the core muscles, including the abdominals, obliques, and supporting muscles that help support the spine and minimize the chances of injury.

Additionally, a study[65] published in the Journal of Physical Therapy Science found that walking on a treadmill at an incline can significantly increase core muscle activation, making it a great option for individuals looking to build core strength.

---

[64] https://www.ncbi.nlm.nih.gov/pmc/articles/PMC5873977/
[65] https://pubmed.ncbi.nlm.nih.gov/28532873/

Increases your bone density

Walking may also aid increase bone density, which is essential for maintaining a healthy spine.

[Studies](#)[66] have shown that weight-bearing workouts like walking on a treadmill can raise the density of your bones and minimize the chances of developing osteoporosis. Regular treadmill walking may also strengthen the muscles and ligaments surrounding the spine, reducing the chances of injury even further.

Promotes overall fitness

Finally, walking is a great way to promote overall fitness, which can positively impact spine health.

Regular exercise can help reduce inflammation, improve circulation, and minimize the chances of developing chronic health conditions such as diabetes, heart disease, and obesity. By promoting overall fitness, treadmill walking can help support spine health and minimize the chances of developing spine-related problems.

Now that you know the power of walking in boosting your spine health, it is time to get on the treadmill and work on a healthier and stronger spine.

---

[66] https://www.ncbi.nlm.nih.gov/pmc/articles/PMC6323511/

Let's move on to the next chapter and learn about the importance of having adequate rest and how it contributes to your spine health.

Chapter 5: The Power of Rest in Healing the Spine

When seeking to heal from a spine injury, most people focus on physical therapy, medication, and surgery options. While these are all important aspects of treatment, rest is an often overlooked factor.

The power of rest is not something you can underestimate when it comes to healing the spine. In fact, proper rest is essential because it gives your spine the time and space it needs to recover fully.

This chapter will explore the many benefits of rest for the spine, including how it can speed up healing, reduce pain and inflammation, and improve overall spinal health.

So, sit back, relax, and discover the transformative power of rest in healing your spine.

The Concept of Anabolism and Its Connection to Rest

Anabolism is the process of building up molecules in the body. It is the opposite of catabolism, which is the process of breaking down molecules.

Anabolism is important for healing because it allows the body to create new tissue to replace damaged or injured tissue. When your spine suffers an injury, anabolism plays a critical role in the spine healing process by helping repair and rebuild damaged cells and tissues.

During the healing process, your body will produce new proteins and cells to replace the damaged ones. This requires a lot of energy and resources, which makes proper nutrition and rest essential for anabolic support.

Adequate rest allows your body to focus its energy on repairing and rebuilding damaged tissues; proper nutrition provides the necessary building blocks (such as proteins, amino acids, and vitamins) for anabolism to occur.

How Does Rest Promote Anabolism?

To understand the role of rest in healing your spine, let's look at the various ways it promotes anabolism:

Promotes protein synthesis

Resting after a spine injury can boost anabolism by promoting protein synthesis. This process helps repair and rebuild the damaged tissues.

Studies[67] have shown that resting after exercise promotes protein synthesis by activating certain signaling pathways that stimulate muscle growth and repair.

Increases growth hormone levels

Resting after a spine injury can boost anabolism by increasing growth hormone levels. Growth hormone is a hormone that stimulates growth and repair in the body.

Studies[68] have shown that sleep and rest can increase growth hormone levels, which can help to promote healing and recovery from injuries.

---

[67] https://pubmed.ncbi.nlm.nih.gov/23717209
[68] https://pubmed.ncbi.nlm.nih.gov/11869601/

Reduces stress hormone levels

Resting after a spine injury can also reduce stress hormone levels in the body, which can help promote healing.

[Research][69] shows that stress hormones like cortisol can inhibit anabolism and protein synthesis, making it harder for the body to repair and rebuild damaged tissues. Resting and reducing stress can help lower cortisol levels and promote anabolism.

Enhances immune function

Resting after a spine injury can also boost anabolism by enhancing immune function. The immune system plays a crucial role in healing and recovery from injuries.

[Research][70] has proven that resting can help enhance immune function by reducing stress and inflammation in the body. This, in turn, can help promote anabolism and aid in the healing process.

Increases blood flow

Resting after a spine injury can also boost anabolism by increasing blood flow to the injured area. Blood carries

---

[69] https://pubmed.ncbi.nlm.nih.gov/15750272/
[70] https://www.ncbi.nlm.nih.gov/pmc/articles/PMC3256323/

nutrients, oxygen, and other essential molecules that promote healing and recovery.

Research[71] shows that resting can help increase blood flow to the injured area, which can help promote anabolism and facilitate healing.

Promotes tissue repair

Resting after a spine injury can also promote anabolism by promoting tissue repair.

Scientific studies[72] have shown that when the body is at rest, it can focus its energy on repairing and rebuilding damaged tissues, which can help promote anabolism and rocket fuel the healing process.

Improves sleep quality

Rest improves the body's circadian rhythm, leading to better sleep quality.

Sleep is a vital component of anabolism, and studies have shown that sleep deprivation can negatively impact muscle protein synthesis, leading to slower healing times. Resting and getting adequate sleep can help boost anabolism and promote healing.

---

[71] https://www.ncbi.nlm.nih.gov/pmc/articles/PMC4376353/
[72] https://www.ncbi.nlm.nih.gov/pmc/articles/PMC3896743/

Reduces stress

Rest and relaxation can help reduce stress levels, and, as you know, stress can negatively impact anabolism. Stress hormones like cortisol can inhibit muscle growth and repair, slowing healing times.

Resting and engaging in relaxation techniques like deep breathing, meditation, and yoga can help lower stress levels and promote anabolism.

Allows for nutrient absorption

During rest, the body's digestive system is less active; this reduced activity allows for better nutrient absorption.

Adequate nutrient intake is essential for anabolism and healing. Resting after a meal can help the body absorb nutrients more efficiently, which can support healing processes.

Clearly, rest plays a huge role in spine regeneration and healing. But how do you get enough rest? Let's find out.

How to Ensure Adequate Rest for Spine Regeneration

Here are a few tips to help you get enough rest to promote spine healing:

Prioritize sleep

Getting enough sleep is essential for overall health and well-being. It is especially important when it comes to spinal healing and regeneration.

During sleep, the body is in a rested state; this rest allows cellular repair and regeneration to take place. When you prioritize sleep and aim for 7-9 hours of uninterrupted rest each night, it gives your body the time it needs to repair and regenerate the tissues in your spine.

To help ensure you get a good night's rest, try establishing a consistent sleep routine, avoid caffeine and alcohol before bed, create a relaxing sleep environment, and use relaxation techniques such as meditation or deep breathing exercises to help you fall asleep more easily.

Limiting exposure to electronics and blue light in the hours leading up to bedtime may also be helpful because this light wavelength can disrupt the body's natural sleep-wake cycle and make it harder to fall asleep.

By making sleep a priority and taking steps to ensure you get enough of it, you can help support the healing and regeneration of your spine.

Use a comfortable mattress

Sleeping on a comfortable mattress is essential for getting enough rest and promoting spine healing and regeneration. When selecting a mattress, consider your sleep preferences and spine condition.

A firm mattress may be suitable if you have a history of back pain, as it provides more support for the spine. A softer mattress may be more comfortable for individuals who sleep on their side, as it can help relieve pressure points.

However, it is important to choose a mattress that strikes a balance between support and comfort. You should also ensure your pillow provides adequate support for your neck and head to maintain proper spinal alignment while sleeping.

Remember that a good quality mattress is an investment in your health and well-being, making it worth the expense.

Take breaks during the day

Incorporating regular breaks into your daily routine can be one of the most effective ways to promote spine healing and regeneration.

When you sit or stand for long periods, the pressure on your spine increases, which can cause discomfort and even lead to injury. This pressure can also restrict blood flow to the spine, making it difficult for the body to deliver the nutrients and oxygen needed for healing and regeneration.

Frequent breaks throughout the day can help alleviate this pressure and improve blood flow to your spine. This increased blood flow can help deliver essential nutrients and oxygen to the injured area, promoting healing and regeneration. Breaks can also help reduce tension and strain on the back muscles and contribute to faster healing.

There are many ways to incorporate breaks into your daily routine. For example, you can take short walks, stretch, or do light exercises during your break time. If you work at a desk, you can try standing up and moving around for a few minutes every hour or use a standing desk to reduce how much time you spend sitting. Taking regular breaks can also be an effective way to reduce stress levels, which can positively impact your overall health and well-being.

Practice good posture

Practicing good posture is crucial to ensuring adequate rest for your spine to heal and regenerate. Poor posture can cause undue pressure on your spine, leading to pain and discomfort. By being mindful of your posture throughout the day, you can reduce this pressure and allow your spine to heal.

When sitting, ensure your back is straight and your feet are flat on the floor. Avoid crossing your legs or slouching forward because this can strain your lower back.

When standing, distribute your weight evenly on both feet and keep your shoulders back and your chin parallel to the ground. Additionally, consider investing in ergonomic chairs or standing desks to support good posture.

With practice, good posture can become a habit and help to promote spine health in the long run.

Practice stress reduction techniques

Stress is known to have negative effects on our bodies, and it can also contribute to back pain and slow down the healing process. When we experience stress, our body releases stress hormones such as cortisol and adrenaline. These hormones can increase inflammation and tension in our back and neck muscles, further exacerbating pain and delaying healing.

Practicing stress reduction techniques can be a simple yet effective way to promote spine healing and regeneration. Deep breathing, meditation, and mindfulness are all great ways to reduce stress and promote relaxation.

Deep breathing, for instance, involves drawing slow, deep breaths in through your nose and out through your mouth. This can help slow down your heart rate, lower blood pressure, and reduce muscle tension, which can help ease back pain.

Similarly, meditation and mindfulness can help reduce stress and improve your mental and emotional well-being. You can start practicing for a few minutes each day and then increase the duration gradually as you become more comfortable with the techniques.

By incorporating stress reduction techniques into your daily routine, you can help to reduce the negative effects of stress on your spine and promote healing and regeneration.

Listen to your body

Listening to your body is crucial to promoting spine healing and regeneration.

When your body is injured, it requires more rest and recovery time to heal properly. When you push yourself too hard, you risk exacerbating your injury or delaying the healing process. Pay attention to any pain or discomfort in your back and adjust your activities or routine accordingly.

For example, if you experience discomfort after sitting for an extended period, try taking a break to stretch or walk around. If you notice that a certain activity or exercise aggravates your back pain, avoid it until your spine has had a chance to heal.

By listening to your body and taking a gentle, loving-kindness approach to your daily activities, you can help ensure your body gets the rest it needs for your spine to heal and regenerate.

Using these tips will give your body the rest it needs to heal and regenerate a healthier and stronger spine.

Conclusion

Hopefully, you now understand what it takes to have a healthy and strong spine. By incorporating the tips we have discussed, a healthy diet, exercise, staying hydrated, and getting proper rest, you will enjoy the benefits of having a strong and healthy spine.

Remember to consult your doctor before making any major lifestyle changes, especially if you already have other underlying medical complications.